CHAIR
FOR SE
OVER 70

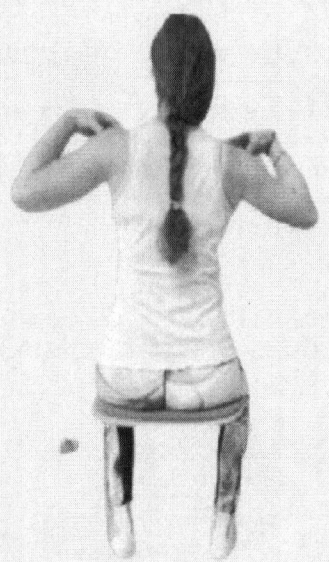

The Ultimate Guide To Help You Improve Your
Flexibility, Strength, and Body Balance With
These Mindful Yoga Exercise

Joyce L. Clark

All rights reserved. No part of this publication may be reproduced, distributed, or transmitted in any form or by any means, including photocopying, recording, or other electronic or mechanical methods, without the prior written permission of the publisher, except in the case of brief quotations embodied in critical reviews and certain other noncommercial uses permitted by copyright law.

Copyright © (Joyce L. Clark), (2023).

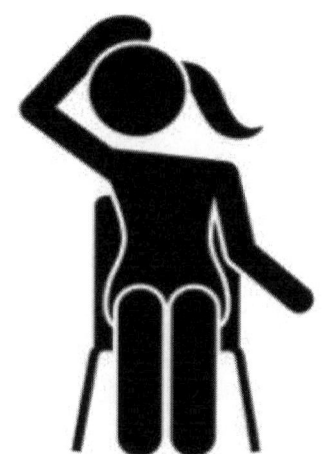

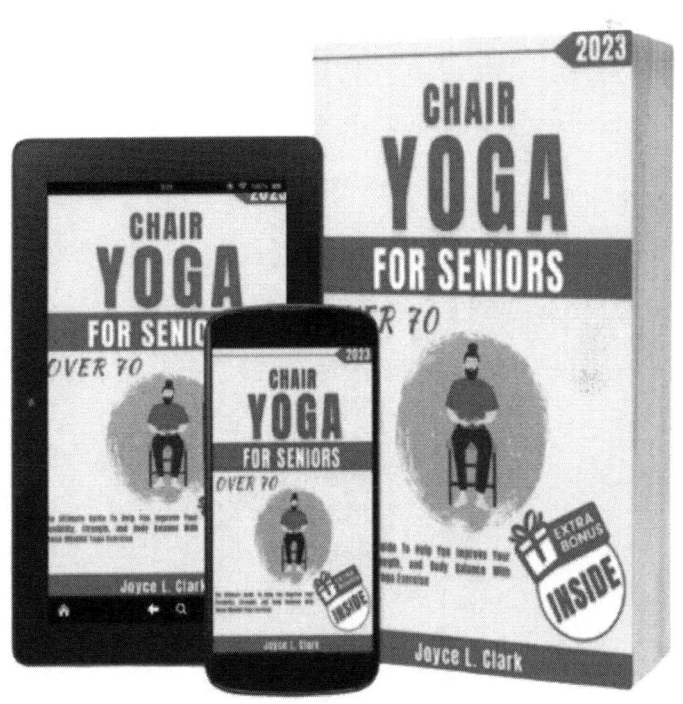

BONUS (COMPLEMENTARY BOOK FOR MY AMAZING READERS)

Thank you for buying this book and I hope that this book will be your guiding **ANGEL!**

To show my appreciation, I am offering you a book which will help you stay healthy while practicing your workout.

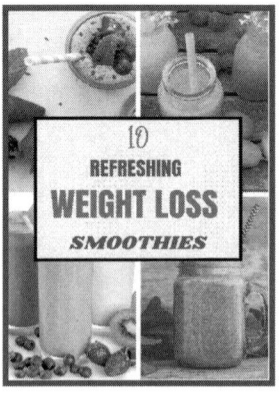

To **CLAIM** This **BONUS**, Follow The Step By Step Guide Available At The "**BONUS SECTION**" Of This Book.

Table Of Contents

INTRODUCTION...8
    Inspiring Story.. 8
    About The Book....................................10
    A Letter From The "Author".................11

CHAPTER ONE....................................... 14
    Understanding Chair Yoga....................14
    How To Incorporate Yoga Into Your Daily Routine.. 18
    Do's And Don't For Practicing Chair Yoga As A Seniors...............................22
    The Best Four (4) Breathing Technique To Master While Practicing Chair Yoga As A Senior..26

CHAPTER TWO.. 32
    Equipment Needed For Chair Yoga.......32
    How To Warm Up Before Starting Your Chair Yoga Exercises............................34
    How To Cool Down After Finishing Your Chair Yoga Exercises............................36
    The Body Protection Tips You Should Master While Working Out...................39

CHAPTER THREE.................................. 42
Simple Poses For Your Daily Routine... 42
  1. Easy Pose.............................. 42
  2. Triangle Pose........................ 44
  3. Warrior Pose.......................... 46
  4. Mountain Pose...................... 48
  5. Standing Poses..................... 51
  6. Half Moon Pose..................... 54
  7. Chair Eagle Pose................... 56
  8. Cat/Cow Pose........................ 58
  9. Child's Pose.......................... 60
  10. Relaxation Pose................... 62
  11. Bridge Pose......................... 64
  12. Cool-Down Poses................ 67
  13. Legs Up the Wall Pose........ 68

CHAPTER FOUR.............................. 72
The Seven (7) Best Chair Yoga Poses 72
  1. Chair Chest Opener.............. 72
  2. Forward Fold........................ 74
  3. Side Bends........................... 77
  4. Neck Stretches..................... 79
  5. Backbend............................. 82
  6. Seated Twist........................ 84

INTROD[UCTION]

Inspiring Story

Ava was a 72-year-old la[dy who was] active. She had been a da[ncer and] still liked walking and tr[ekking. She] had been feeling stiff an[d realized] that she needed to do so[mething for] flexibility, strength, and [balance but didn't] know where to start.

Ava started surfing the i[nternet and came] across a book called "C[hair Yoga for Seniors] Over 70". The chair yoga [in the book was] particularly intended for p[eople who couldn't] undertake standard yoga [poses. The poses] are adjusted so that they [may be performed] in a chair. Ava was so inte[rested that she decided to] give it a try.

7. Spinal Twist.................. 86

The Six (6) Breathing Yoga Exercises For Seniors..................89
1. Deep Breathing................ 89
3. Nadi Shodhana................. 91
4. Meditation for Seniors....... 94
5. Mindfulness Meditation....... 97
6. Guided Meditation............ 99

Sixteen (16) Chair Yoga Cardio Exercise For Weight Loss.................103
1. Chair Yoga Nidra............. 103
2. Chair arm circles............ 106
3. Chair shoulder shrugs........ 108
4. Chair chest openers.......... 111
5. Chair twists................. 113
6. Chair arm rises.............. 115
7. Chair leg raises............. 117
8. Chair knee tucks............. 119
9. Chair hip circles............ 122
10. Chair hamstring stretch..... 124
11. Chair calf stretch.......... 126
12. Chair squat................. 128
13. Chair lunge................. 131
14. Chair push-ups.............. 133

15. Chair plank

16. Chair mou[n]

CHAPTER FIVE

How To Avoid

Benefits Of A

How To Make

Will Increase Y

Your Inflamma

Lifestyle..........

CONCLUSION..

BONUS SECT

After she discovered chair yoga and began practicing the positions at home. At first, it was challenging. Her muscles were stiff, and she had problems balancing. But she persisted at it, and eventually, she began to notice progress.

After a few weeks, Ava noted that she was feeling more flexible. She could reach her toes more easily, and she wasn't as stiff when she stood up from a chair. She was also stronger. She could carry groceries without feeling exhausted, and she wasn't as quickly winded as she walked.

But the most notable change was in her balance. She no longer felt shaky, and she was less likely to tumble. She was so thrilled with the effects of chair yoga that she promoted it to all of her friends.

Ava continued to practice chair yoga for many years. She ultimately grew so flexible and powerful that she was able to complete several of the standard yoga positions. She also began teaching chair yoga lessons to other seniors in her neighborhood. She was very pleased that she had discovered chair yoga, and she knew that it had made a tremendous impact in her life.

Welcome To This Book "Chair Yoga For Seniors Over 70"

About The Book

This book offers a complete guide to practicing chair yoga for seniors especially who are over the age of 70.

It gives step-by-step directions for over 40 postures that can be done in a chair, as well as information on the advantages of chair yoga for seniors.

This book is for anybody who is over the age of 70 who wants to enhance their flexibility, strength, balance, and general health.

It is also a terrific resource for persons with mobility challenges or impairments.

This book can benefit you in the following ways:

- Learn how to execute chair yoga postures safely and successfully.
- Improve your flexibility, strength, balance, and general wellness.
- Reduce pain and stiffness.
- Improve your mood and lessen stress.
- Increase your energy levels.
- Improve your sleep.
- Promote relaxation and mindfulness.

A Letter From The "Author"

I aim to utilize this book to assist you to live healthier, happier, and more active lives. I feel that chair yoga is a terrific approach to attain these aims, and I hope that this book will motivate you to give it a try.

I also want to utilize this book to increase awareness of the advantages of chair yoga for seniors. Many people are not aware that chair yoga is a safe and effective approach to enhance their health, and I hope that this book will help to alter that.

I am happy to share this book with the world and assist as many people as possible experience the advantages of chair yoga.

I Hope That You Like This Book

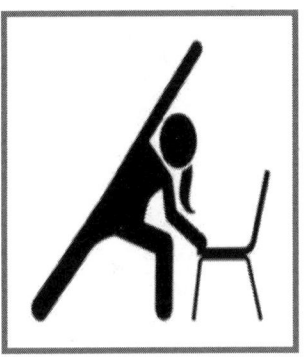

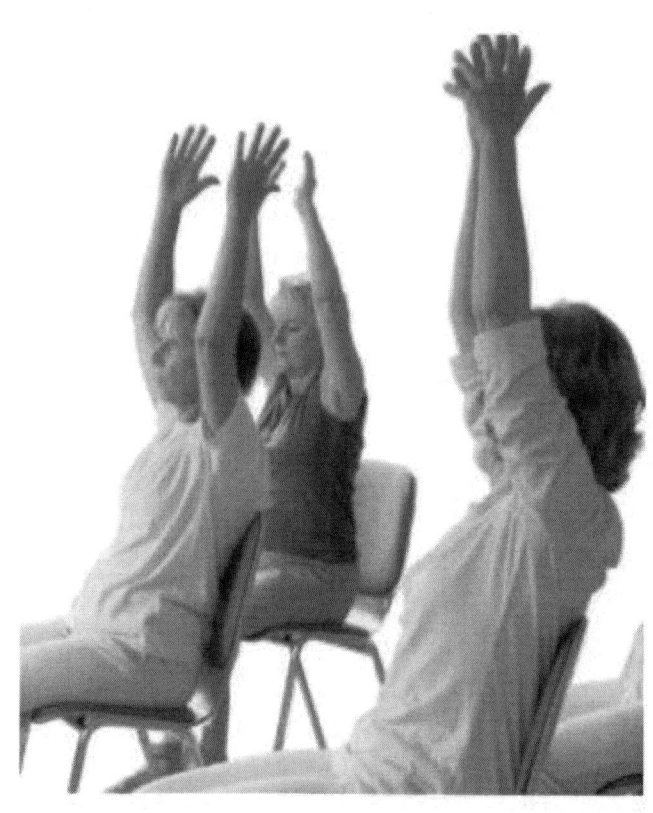

CHAPTER ONE

Understanding Chair Yoga

If you work in an office or drive a bus, there's no getting past the reality that you're on your seat more than you're on your feet. But medical professionals believe adding lots of activity to your day is crucial to optimum health. That's where chair yoga postures come in.

Chair yoga is a style of yoga that is done while sitting in a chair. It is an excellent choice for persons who are unable to practice regular yoga positions due to injury, sickness, or age. Chair yoga can also be a wonderful approach to teach yoga to persons who are new to it.

Chair yoga poses adjusted for a sitting position have proven a benefit for persons who have injuries, reduced mobility, or physical limitations. But even the healthiest person may do asana in a chair to stretch tight muscles, keep your joints supple, and aid enhanced blood flow.

Chair yoga postures are meant to be gentle and accessible to everyone. They emphasize on stretching and strengthening the main muscular groups, as well as enhancing balance and flexibility.

The Benefits Of Chair Yoga For Seniors:

1. Increased flexibility and range of motion: As we age, our muscles and joints tend to become rigid and inflexible. Chair yoga may assist to increase flexibility and range of motion by gently stretching and strengthening the muscles. This may make it simpler to do daily tasks, such as getting up and down from a chair, walking, and dressing.

2. Improved balance and coordination: Balance and coordination might diminish with aging, increasing the risk of falls. Chair yoga may assist to improve balance and coordination by pushing the body in a safe and regulated setting. This may assist to lower the risk of falls and enhance general mobility.

3. Increased muscular strength: Chair yoga may help to strengthen muscle strength, which can assist to improve posture, decrease discomfort, and raise energy levels.

4. Reduced stress and anxiety: Chair yoga may help to reduce stress and anxiety by fostering relaxation and awareness. The slow, controlled movements and concentrated breathing of chair yoga may assist to soothe the mind and body.

5. Improved mood and sleep quality: Chair yoga may assist to enhance mood and sleep quality by lowering stress and anxiety. Yoga may also assist to produce endorphins, which have mood-boosting benefits.

6. Reduced discomfort: Chair yoga may help to relieve pain linked with illnesses such as arthritis, back pain, and headaches. The mild stretching and strengthening exercises may assist to increase flexibility and range of motion, which can alleviate pain and stiffness.

7. Improved overall health and well-being: Chair yoga may assist to promote overall health and well-being by boosting physical fitness, mental health, and relaxation. It is a low-impact sport that can be enjoyed by individuals of all fitness levels, making it a fantastic alternative for seniors.

Chair yoga is a safe and effective approach to develop your flexibility, balance, strength, and relieve tension and discomfort. **Why not give it a try!**

If you want to get the most out of chair yoga, you need to follow these steps:

- Find a comfy chair that you can sit in for lengthy amounts of time.
- Wear loose-fitting attire that will enable you to move freely.

- Start with a few easy positions and progressively add more as you gain stronger and more flexible.
- Listen to your body and don't push yourself too much.
- Take breaks as required.
- Breathe deeply during the exercise.

With a little practice, you will be astonished at how much you can gain from chair yoga.

How To Incorporate Yoga Into Your Daily Routine

Incorporating yoga into your daily routine can be a game-changer for both your physical and emotional well-being. The ancient discipline of yoga has been around for thousands of years and provides a broad variety of advantages that can help you enjoy a more balanced, healthy, and meaningful life.

From developing flexibility and strength to lowering tension and anxiety, yoga may help you reach a feeling of quiet and tranquility that is hard to find in today's fast-paced world. But with so many various kinds and techniques of yoga, it may be tough to know where to start.

How can you make yoga a regular part of your everyday routine? How do you choose the best type of yoga for you? And how do you keep yourself motivated and on track?

If you're new to yoga, or if you're wanting to include it into your daily routine, you need this tips:

1. Start small and be consistent. You don't have to complete an hour-long yoga session every day. Just a few minutes of practice may make a tremendous impact. Start with 5 or 10 minutes a day, and gradually increase the duration as you get more comfortable.

2. Find a time and location that works for you. Some individuals like to do yoga first thing in the morning, while others prefer to do it at night. Find a time that you're most likely to keep to and make sure you have a peaceful spot to practice where you won't be disturbed.

3. Find a type of yoga that you appreciate. There are many various forms of yoga, so it's vital to select one that you find pleasurable and that matches your fitness level. Some prominent styles are Hatha, Vinyasa, and Iyengar.

4. Use props. If you're new to yoga, or if you have any ailments, you may wish to utilize props like blocks, straps, or blankets. Props may help you get into the postures securely and comfortably.

5. Listen to your body. Don't push yourself too much. If you're suffering discomfort, cease the stance and rest. Yoga is about listening to your body and recognising its boundaries.

6. Make it a habit. The key to integrating yoga into your everyday routine is to make it a habit. Just like brushing your teeth, aim to practice yoga at the same time each day.

Include these methods into your everyday routine, if you want to get the most out of your exercise.

1. Wake up with yoga. A few sun salutations or a mild yoga sequence will help you wake up your body and mind and start your day off correctly.

2. Take a yoga break at work. If you have a few minutes, you may practice some easy yoga positions at your desk or in a conference room.

3. Practice yoga before bed. Yoga may help you relax and unwind before bed, which can enhance your sleep quality.

4. Incorporate yoga into your fitness programme. You may practice some yoga positions before or after your exercise to increase your flexibility and range of motion.

5. Make yoga a family activity. Yoga is a terrific way to get the entire family active and having fun.

No matter how you include yoga into your daily practice, the main target is to be consistent. The more you practice, the more you'll receive the advantages of yoga.

Do's And Don't For Practicing Chair Yoga As A Seniors

Just because you've reached your Golden Years doesn't mean you can't still engage in yoga. In fact, even 15 to 35 minutes of low impact stretches and postures can do wonders for the mobility and flexibility of elders.

Too many older folks assume that yoga is too tough or demanding and avoid taking part, although nothing could be farther from the truth. It's just as vital for seniors to keep active as it is for everyone in order to remain healthy and happy. Yoga may be a vital component of a sensible exercise plan for seniors and one of the most popular routines today is Chair Yoga. This is something you can do in the comfort and privacy of your own home, as there is no need to travel to a yoga studio or gym to practice Chair Yoga.

But there are several Do's And Don't you should know when performing chair yoga as a senior. These are as follows:

Dos:

- Find a comfy chair with a backrest that supports your spine.
- Start softly and progressively raise the intensity of your practice as you get more comfortable.
- Listen to your body and stop if you experience any discomfort.

- Focus on your breathing and relax your muscles as you move.
- Be careful of your alignment and make sure you are not exerting too much pressure on any one section of your body.
- Stay hydrated by drinking lots of water before, during, and after your practice.
- Find a supportive group of individuals who can inspire and motivate you.

Don'ts:

- Push yourself too hard.
- Force yourself into any stance that is unpleasant.
- Hold a stance for too long if it is causing discomfort.
- Do not practice if you are feeling ill.
- Compare yourself to others.
- Be frightened to seek assistance.

Practicing these extra chair yoga tips would help you get the most out of your exercise as a senior.

- Wear comfortable attire that enables you to move freely.
- Remove any jewelry that might get trapped on your clothes or the chair.
- Warm up your body before commencing your practice with some simple stretches.
- Cool down your body after your session with some deep breathing and relaxation techniques.
- Practice consistently to gain the maximum advantages from chair yoga.

The Best Four (4) Breathing Technique To Master While Practicing Chair Yoga As A Senior

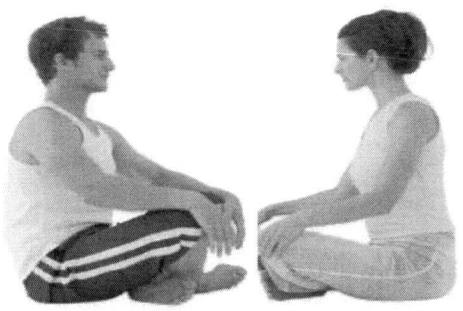

Starting chair yoga or any kind of exercises will not be complete if you did not master the acts of breathing. Breathing is good for our health and here I will provide you with 4 breathing methods that you can learn and perfect when Practicing chair yoga as a senior:

1. Diaphragmatic breathing. This is the most frequent form of breathing and includes breathing from your diaphragm, the muscle that divides your chest from your belly.

To practice diaphragmatic breathing, sit in a comfortable chair with your feet flat on the floor and your back straight. Place one hand on your chest and the other on your stomach. As you inhale, breathe deeply such that your stomach rises and your chest remains relatively steady. As you exhale, breathe out gently such that your stomach descends and your chest remains reasonably steady.

2. Alternate nostril breathing. This is a soothing breathing method that helps to balance the body's energy. To practice alternate nostril breathing, sit in a comfortable chair with your legs crossed and your back straight.

Close your right nostril with your right thumb and inhale softly through your left nose. Hold your breath for a few seconds, then exhale gently through your right nostril. Repeat this cycle for 5-10 breaths, then swap sides and repeat.

3. Ujjayi breathing. This is a strong breathing technique that helps to boost attention and concentration. It is a method that helps you to quiet your mind by concentrating on your breath.

This method helps you overcome ideas that may perhaps distract you from your meditative state.

It's the most popular kind of pranayama (breath control) employed during asana (body posture/pose) practices.

How To Conduct Ujjayi Breathing

As you inhale and exhale:

- Keep your mouth closed.
- Constrict your throat to the extent that your breathing creates a rushing noise, almost like snoring.
- Control your breath using your diaphragm.

- Keep your inhalations and exhalations similar in length.
- This may be peaceful and balanced.

At first, it may seem like you're not receiving enough air, but the technique should grow simpler with repetition.

4. Kapalbhati breathing. This is a cleansing breathing method that helps to eliminate toxins from the body. It is a highly strong breathing technique that not only helps you lose weight but also puts your complete system into a perfect equilibrium.

To practice this techniques, you will have to follow this process:

- Sit comfortably with your spine erect. Place your hands on the knees with palms open to the heavens. Kapalbhati Pranayama

- Take a big breath in.

- As you breathe, pull your stomach. Pull your navel back towards the spine. Do as much as you comfortably can. You may keep your right hand on the stomach to feel the abdominal muscles tense.

- As you relax the navel and abdomen, the air pours into your lungs spontaneously.

- Take 20 such breaths to complete one round of KapalBhati Pranayama.

- After finishing the cycle, rest with your eyes closed and analyze the feelings in your body.

- Do two additional rounds of KapalBhati Pranayama.

Tips For Following The Workouts

- The exhale in the Skull Shining Breathing method is energetic and strong. So, simply throw out your breath.

- Don't worry about inhaling. The instant you relax your abdominal muscles, inhalation will proceed automatically.

- Keep your concentration on breathing out.

- Practice this method at home on an empty stomach.

CHAPTER TWO

Equipment Needed For Chair Yoga

Though chair yoga is a low-risk and low-impact type of exercise, you need to make sure you have the correct equipment to avoid injuries and to get the most out of your practice.

The equipment required for chair yoga is simple and can be bought at any home or sporting goods shops. Here are the important equipments you need:

1. An armless, sturdy chair: A chair with arms might make it difficult to accomplish some of the positions, so it's preferable to use a chair without them. The chair should also be sturdy so that you don't wobble or fall over.

2. A flat, level surface: The chair should be positioned on a smooth, level surface so that you don't lose your equilibrium.

3. **Flexible, comfortable attire:** You'll want to wear clothing that enables you to move freely and comfortably. Avoid wearing anything excessively tight or confining.

4. **Space to completely extend your limbs:** You'll need adequate space to fully stretch your limbs in the positions. Make sure you have an adequate area around you so that you don't crash into anything.

Optional:

- **Yoga blocks:** Yoga blocks may be used to support your body in some of the positions.
- **Yoga straps:** Yoga straps may be used to assist you reach your hands behind your back or over your head.
- **Blanket:** A blanket may be used to give additional padding or warmth.

It is a good idea to start chair yoga with a simple chair and a few basic props. As you feel more comfortable, you may add additional props and push yourself with more complex positions.

How To Warm Up Before Starting Your Chair Yoga Exercises

When you practice chair yoga, warm-ups are vital. Warming up for any physical activity minimizes injuries and boosts performance. Chair yoga warm-ups only take a few minutes, so don't neglect them. After just five to ten minutes of warm-up activities, blood flow to muscles rises by up to 75 percent.

It's common in yoga to start with particular warm-ups, typically termed sun salutations or vinyasa flows. Vinyasa means to connect breath to movement. Greeting the sun by moving the body with breath helps put us in a right mental state to flow more freely and move with greater ease.

Think of warm-up flows as movement meditations. Often, we go about our day aimlessly. When we take time to relate our breath to our activity, our mind and body become linked, and we have a much clearer view on our day. We also start to live our lives with greater purpose and clarity. It's astonishing to imagine that just a few focused motions can mean so much.

Warm-up

- Start by sitting up straight in your chair with your feet flat on the floor. Take a few deep breaths to bring your awareness to your body.
- Gently move your shoulders forward and back, then side to side.
- Reach your arms aloft and then down to your sides.
- Do some neck stretches by gently nodding your head forth and back, then side to side.
- Stand up and perform some mild leg swings.

- You may also attempt some easy yoga positions like cat/cow pose or sitting twists.

The purpose of the warm-up is to raise your heart rate, blood flow, and range of motion. This will assist you avoid injuries and make your yoga practice more pleasurable.

How To Cool Down After Finishing Your Chair Yoga Exercises

At every end of a more rigorous or physically taxing yoga practice, take the time to cool down with some hip openers, reclining twists, and passive inversions. These postures may also stand on their own when you want to relax your body, but you'll go deeper when you're warmed up.

You can also use this programme as a cooldown after other types of exercise. Cooldowns assist avoid lightheadedness or dizziness that may develop if you train at greater intensities but stop quickly without allowing blood flow to return to normal.

A decent cooldown can also function as a segue between your exercise and a return to your everyday routines, soothing you and concluding the session on a peaceful note.

The best tips on how to cool down in the right way.

Cool-down

- After your yoga session, spend a few minutes to chill down. This will allow your body to recuperate and avoid muscular discomfort.
- You may perform some mild stretches or yoga exercises.
- It is also useful to take several deep breaths and calm your body.

- The cool-down helps to restore your body back to its resting condition and drain out any toxins.

Want to practice some of the particular chair yoga positions that will help you stay warm-up or even help you cool-down? **Try these exercises.**

Warm-up:

- Chair cat/cow pose
- Seated twists
- Chair arm circles

Cool-down:

- Child's posture
- Seated forward bend
- Neck rolls

The Body Protection Tips You Should Master While Working Out

Whether you're a casual fitness enthusiast or hard-core gym geek, being hurt while working out doesn't have to be an unavoidable part of life.

The best 7 strategies to help you avoid injuries while exercising:

1. Listen to your body. Don't push yourself too hard or beyond your limitations. If you experience discomfort, cease the position and relax.

2. Warm up before you start. This will assist to avoid injury. A nice warm-up may involve some mild stretching and marching in place.

3. Cool down when you finish. This will enable your body to recuperate. A good cool-down could include some gentle stretching and deep breathing.

4. Use a supporting chair. A robust chair with a backrest can assist to protect your back and spine.

5. Don't lock your joints. This might put stress on your muscles and joints.

6. Breathe deeply throughout the exercise. This will help to oxygenate your muscles and prevent fatigue.

7. Stay hydrated. Drink lots of water before, during, and after your exercise.

Here are some more guidelines for safeguarding your body particularly during chair yoga:

- Use a chair that is the perfect height for you. Your feet should lie level on the floor and your knees should be slightly bent.
- Don't put too much weight on your arms. If you need to, use a strap or cloth to assist you balance.

- Be cautious while executing positions that entail twisting or bending. These stances may put stress on your back and neck.
- If you have any health concerns, consult your doctor before beginning chair yoga.

Chair yoga is an effective method to get a workout without placing too much stress on your body. By following these suggestions, you can be able to assist and safeguard your body by getting the most out of your practice.

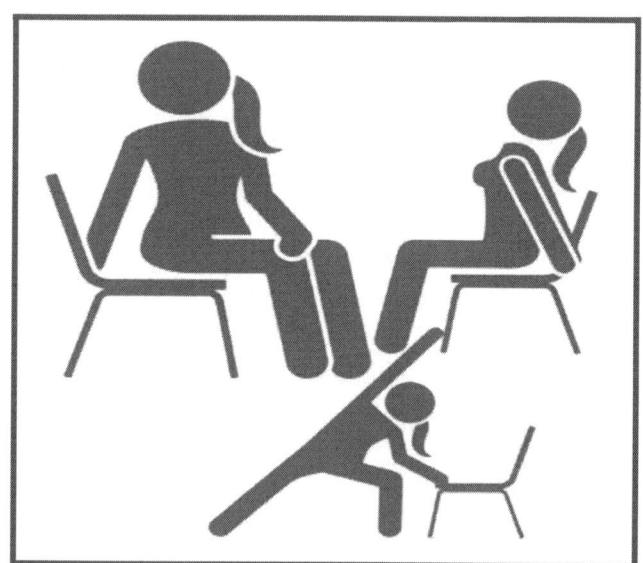

CHAPTER THREE

Simple Poses For Your Daily Routine

1. Easy Pose

Chair Easy posture (also known as Sukhasana) is a basic yoga posture that may be done by individuals of all fitness levels. It is a terrific technique to improve your posture, decrease tension, and boost your attention.

Follow these Instructions to help you accomplish Chair Easy Pose:

- Sit on a chair with your feet flat on the floor.
- Place your hands on your thighs, palms down.
- Relax your shoulders and neck.
- Lengthen your spine by pulling your tailbone down and your head up.

- Close your eyes and concentrate on your breath.
- Stay in this stance for 5-10 breaths, or as long as you feel comfortable.
- To get out of the posture, just open your eyes and stand up.

Tips to help you perform Chair Easy Pose in the right way:

- If you have tight hips, you might tuck a wrapped towel or blanket beneath your knees.
- If you experience lower back discomfort, you may tilt forward slightly.
- If you experience neck ache, you may lay your forehead on your hands.
- If you are feeling dizzy or lightheaded, get out of the posture immediately.

Advantages of practicing Chair Easy Pose:

Improves posture Reduces stress Increases focus Relieves back pain Improves digestion Boosts energy levels Promotes relaxation

If you are new to yoga, Chair Easy Pose is a terrific place to start. It is a basic stance that can be done anywhere, and it offers numerous advantages for your health and well-being.

2. Triangle Pose

Follow these Instructions to help you accomplish Chair Triangle Pose:

- Stand next to a chair with your right side closest to the chair.
- Plant your feet approximately 3 to 4 feet apart.
- Turn your right foot so your toes point toward the chair and plant your left foot at a 45-degree angle.

- Inhale and bring your arms up to shoulder height, parallel to the floor.
- Exhale and bend forward from your hip joint, bringing your left arm down toward your left foot. You may rest your left hand on your shin or thigh, or on the seat of the chair if you need to.
- Keep your right arm stretching up toward the ceiling, keep your spine long and your core engaged.
- Hold the posture for 5 to 10 breaths, then gently come back to standing.
- Repeat on the opposite side.

Tips to help you perform Chair Triangle Pose in the right way:

- If you have any knee discomfort, you may bend your right knee slightly.
- If you find it difficult to reach your left foot, you might raise your left hand to your hip.

- Don't push the stance if you feel any discomfort.

Advantages of performing the Chair Triangle Pose:

- Improves balance and coordination
- Stretches the hips, shoulders, and spine
- Opens the chest and lungs
- Strengthens the legs and core
- Reduces stress

3. Warrior Pose

Follow these Instructions to help you accomplish Chair Warrior Pose:

- Sit on the edge of a chair with your feet flat on the floor hip-width apart.
- Place your hands on the armrests of the chair, shoulder-width apart.

- Inhale, then as you exhale, straighten your right leg and stretch it out in front of you, maintaining your heel on the floor.
- Turn your body to the right, such that your right shoulder is above your right knee.
- Keep your left leg bowed and your left foot flat on the floor.
- Press down through your feet and elevate your chest, stretching your spine.
- Gaze over your right fingers.
- Hold the posture for 3-5 breaths, then repeat on the opposite side.

Tips to help you perform Chair Warrior Pose in the right way:

- If you feel any discomfort in your knee, bend it more.
- If you can't retain your balance, grip onto the edges of the chair for support.
- Don't push the posture. If you feel any tension in your hips or back, release the position and come back to it later.

Advantages of performing the Chair Warrior Pose:

- Improves balance and coordination
- Strengthens the legs, hips, and core
  Improves flexibility in the hips, spine, and shoulders
- Opens up the chest and lungs
- Reduces stress and anxiety
- Promotes a feeling of peace and well-being

If you're searching for a tough and rewarding yoga posture to add to your practice, the Chair Warrior posture is a good alternative.

4. Mountain Pose

Chair Mountain practice, also known as Chair Tadasana, is a sitting yoga practice that is a modification of the conventional Mountain Pose (Tadasana). It is a fantastic posture for novices and individuals with restricted movement, since it gives support from the chair.

Follow these Instructions to help you accomplish Chair Mountain Pose:

- Sit on the edge of a chair with your feet flat on the floor hip-width apart.
- Place your hands on the sides of the chair, shoulder-width apart.
- Inhale, and stretch your spine from the top of your head to your tailbone.
- Exhale, and tilt your pelvis forward slightly, engage your core, and elevate your chest.
- Keep your shoulders relaxed and low, and your attention ahead.
- Hold the posture for 30 seconds to a minute, inhaling deeply.
- To come out of the posture, inhale, and gently remove your hands off the chair.

Tips to help you perform Chair Mountain Pose in the right way:

- If you feel any discomfort in your knees, drop your hips until you reach a comfortable posture.
- If you find it difficult to retain your equilibrium, you may grab onto the back of the chair.
- As you gain stronger, you may attempt raising your hands off the chair and holding them in prayer posture at your heart center.

Advantages of Chair Mountain Pose include:

- Strengthening the legs, hips, and core Improving balance and coordination
- Lengthening the spine
- Reducing stress and anxiety
- Improving circulation

It is vital to start this exercise cautiously and progressively extend the time of the posture as you feel more comfortable. If you have any health issues, please speak with your doctor before doing yoga.

5. Standing Poses

Follow these Instructions to help you accomplish chair standing poses:

- Sit on a firm chair with your feet flat on the floor hip-width apart.
- Place your hands on the armrests of the chair for support.
- Inhale and straighten your spine, elevating your chest and bringing your shoulders back.
- Exhale and lean forward from your hips, keeping your back straight.
- Reach your arms down towards the floor, keeping your shoulders relaxed.

- Hold for 5 breaths, then gently return to the starting position.

If you are having enough of this exercise, you can go for this alternative chair standing postures which is also good to your body:

- **Chair Warrior Pose:** From a sitting posture, put your hands on the armrests of the chair and raise your right leg up and over your left leg. Rotate your body to the right and stare over your right shoulder. Hold for 5 breaths, then swap sides.

- **Chair Triangle Pose:** From a sitting posture, put your right hand on the armrest of the chair and stretch your left arm out to the side, parallel to the floor. Lean to the left, keeping your back straight and your left shoulder down. Hold for 5 breaths, then swap sides.

- **Chair Tree Pose:** From a sitting posture, raise your right leg up and rest your right foot on the inner of your left thigh. Press down through your feet and plant your hips into the chair. Hold for 5 breaths, then swap sides.

These are just a few examples of chair standing positions. There are many different postures that you may attempt, depending on your fitness level and flexibility. If you are new to yoga, it is usually advisable to start with basic positions and gradually work your way up to more strenuous ones.

Tips to help you perform chair standing poses in the right way:

- Listen to your body and don't push yourself too much.
- If you experience any discomfort, cease the position and relax.
- Focus on your breath and relax your muscles.

- Be patient and consistent in your practice.

With frequent practice, you will start to see and feel the advantages of chair standing postures. You will enhance your balance, flexibility, and strength. You will also decrease stress and boost your mood.

6. Half Moon Pose

Follow these Instructions to help you accomplish Chair Half Moon Pose:

- Stand in front of a chair with your feet hip-width apart and your toes pointed forward.
- Bend your right knee and rest your right forearm on the seat of the chair, directly above your knee.
- Rotate your right thigh outward so that your kneecap is facing straight ahead.
- Extend your left leg behind you, keeping your toes pointed.

- Reach your left arm up above, parallel to the floor.
- Gaze in the direction of your left hand.
- Hold the posture for 5-10 breaths, then repeat on the opposite side.

Tips to help you perform Chair Half Moon Pose in the right way:

- Keep your core engaged throughout the position.
- Don't let your back arch.
- If you feel any discomfort in your knee, bend it further or lay a block beneath your foot.
- If you find it difficult to balance, you may maintain your eyes on a fixed spot in front of you.

Advantages of the Chair Half Moon Pose:

- Improves balance and coordination

- Strengthens the legs, hips, and core Improves flexibility in the hips and spine
- Opens up the chest and shoulders
- Reduces stress and anxiety Improves mood and energy levels

If you are searching for a tough but rewarding yoga practice, the Chair Half Moon practice is a perfect alternative. With consistent practice, you will be shocked at how much your balance, strength, and flexibility develop.

7. Chair Eagle Pose

Follow these Instructions to help you accomplish Chair Eagle Pose:

- Sit up straight on the chair with your feet flat on the floor.
- Cross your right thigh across your left leg, bringing your right foot to rest on the left thigh.

- Cross your right arm across your left arm at the elbow, bringing your hands to contact.
- Hold for 5-10 breaths. Repeat on the opposite side.

Following these basic recommendations can help you practice your chair sitting postures exercises in the right way:

- Start softly and progressively raise the intensity of your practice as you grow stronger.
- Listen to your body and stop if you experience any discomfort.
- Be careful to breathe deeply and evenly during the exercises.
- Focus on your alignment and make sure that your spine is constantly long and your shoulders are relaxed.
- Have fun and enjoy the process!

8. Cat/Cow Pose

Follow these Instructions to help you accomplish Chair Cat/Cow Pose:

- Sit on a firm chair with your feet level on the floor and your back straight.
- Place your hands on your thighs, palms down.
- Inhale, and as you exhale, round your back, tucking your chin into your chest.
- Inhale, and as you exhale, arch your back, elevating your head and chest.
- Repeat steps 3 and 4 for 5-10 breaths.

Tips to help you perform Chair Cat/Cow Pose in the right way:

- Keep your neck long and relaxed.
- Don't push the motions.
- If you feel any discomfort, pause and change your stance.

Advantages of performing the Chair Cat/Cow Pose:

- Improves posture
- Stretches and strengthens the spine
- Relieves back pain Improves flexibility
- Stimulates the abdominal organs
- Calms the mind and body

The Chair Cat/Cow Pose is a gentle technique to stretch and strengthen your spine. It can be done by persons of various ages and fitness levels. It is an effective technique to improve your posture and flexibility, and it may also assist to ease back discomfort.

9. Child's Pose

Follow these Instructions to help you accomplish Chair Child's Pose:

- Sit in a chair with your feet flat on the floor and your knees hip-width apart.

- Lean forward from your hips, keeping your back straight.
- Rest your torso on your thighs, or on a folded blanket if required.
- Let your arms lie at your sides, or stretch them forward and set your palms on the floor in front of you.
- Close your eyes and relax your whole body.
- Breathe deeply and evenly for 5-10 breaths.
- To emerge out of the stance, carefully roll back up to a sitting position.

Here are some tweaks you may apply to the posture if needed:

- If you have tight hips, you may bend your knees more.
- If you experience lower back discomfort, you may position a cushion beneath your knees.

- If you have difficulties reaching the floor, you may lay a block or folded blanket in front of you to rest your hands on.

Advantages of performing Chair Child's Pose:

- Relieves stress and tension
- Improves flexibility in the hips, spine, and shoulders
- Opens the chest and lungs
- Calms the mind and nerve system
- Reduces lower back pain
- Improves circulation
- Promotes relaxation

Chair Child's Pose is an effective technique to release tension, enhance your flexibility, and expand your hips. It is a beginner-friendly position that can be done anywhere, making it a perfect alternative for busy individuals.

10. Relaxation Pose

This stance is a basic and powerful stance that can be done anywhere, even if you are seated in a chair. It is a terrific method to reduce stress and anxiety, and to enhance your general health and well-being.

Follow these Instructions to help you accomplish Chair Relaxation Pose:

- Sit in a chair with your back straight and your feet flat on the floor.
- Close your eyes and take a few deep breaths.
- Place your hands on your thighs, palms down.
- Inhale and gently lean forward, maintaining your back straight.
- Hold for a few seconds, then exhale and return to the beginning position.
- Repeat 3-5 times.

As you perform the position, concentrate on your breath and on relaxing your muscles. You may also choose to envision a serene landscape or setting.

Here are some more techniques for executing the Chair Relaxation Pose:

- If you have any neck or shoulder ache, you may tuck a wrapped towel or blanket behind your neck for support.
- If you are feeling dizzy or lightheaded, discontinue the position and relax.
- You may also execute this stance with your eyes open, if you choose.

Advantages of performing the Chair Relaxation Pose:

- Reduces stress and anxiety
- Improves circulation
- Relieves muscular tension Improves posture
- Boosts energy levels Improves sleep quality
- Promotes relaxation and tranquilly

The Chair Relaxation Pose is a simple and easy technique to enhance your health and well-being. Try it now and see how it makes you feel!

11. Bridge Pose

Follow these Instructions to help you accomplish Chair Bridge Pose:

- Sit in a chair with your feet flat on the floor, hip-width apart.
- Place your hands on the edges of the chair, right above your hips.
- Inhale and push down into your feet and hands, bringing your hips up off the seat of the chair.
- Keep your core engaged and your spine long.
- Hold the posture for 5-10 breaths, then gently descend back down to the seat of the chair.

Tips to help you perform Chair Bridge Pose in the right way:

- If you are new to yoga, you may wish to start with your knees bent. As you grow stronger, you can straighten your knees.
- If you have any back discomfort, be cautious not to arch your back too much. Instead, concentrate on pushing your hips up in a controlled way.
- You may also accomplish this stance without a chair. To do this, lay on your back with your knees bent and your feet flat on the floor. Place your hands on your hips and push down into your feet, bringing your hips up off the floor.

Advantages of practicing the Chair Bridge Pose:

- Strengthens the back muscles, glutes, and hamstrings
- Relieves tightness and weariness in the back

- Improves core strength
- Stretches the chest, neck, and spine
- Opens the lungs
- Calms the brain

The Chair Bridge Pose is an effective technique to develop your back muscles, glutes, and hamstrings. It may also assist to reduce stress and tiredness in your back. If you are searching for a mild technique to enhance your core strength, this is an excellent posture to try.

12. Cool-Down Poses

Here are some chair cool-down positions exercises:

Chair Forward Fold:

- Sit in a chair with your spine straight and feet flat on the floor.
- Hinge forward from the hips and allow your body to collapse between your legs.

- When you can no longer bend any farther, round your spine and sink your head toward the floor.
- Slowly roll up to sitting.

Chair Calf Stretch:

- Sit on a chair with your feet flat on the floor.
- Reach for your toes, or as far as you can comfortably reach.
- Hold the stretch for 30 seconds.
- You may perform these positions in any sequence that you choose. Hold each stance for 30 seconds to 1 minute, or longer if you feel comfortable. Breathe deeply and relax into the stretches.

Tips to help you perform chair cool-down poses in the right way:

- Start with easy exercises and progressively increase the intensity as you warm up.

- Listen to your body and stop if you experience any discomfort.
- Be mindful to breathe deeply throughout the positions.
- Finish with a few minutes of relaxation to let your body recuperate.

13. Legs Up the Wall Pose

This posture is a restorative yoga posture that is simple to execute and has several benefits, including:

- Reducing stress and anxiety
- Improving circulation
- Relieving headaches and migraines
- Reducing edema in the legs and feet
- Improving digestion
- Boosting energy levels
- Relaxing the mind and body

Follow these Instructions to help you accomplish Chair Legs Up the Wall Pose:

- Find a chair that is the correct height for you. You should be able to sit on the chair with your feet flat on the floor and your knees bent at a 90-degree angle.
- Place a yoga mat or blanket behind you.
- Sit in the chair and lean back into the mat or blanket.
- Bend your knees and position your feet flat on the wall, hip-width apart.
- Relax your legs and let them rest against the wall.
- If you feel comfortable, you may shut your eyes and rest your arms at your sides.
- Stay in this stance for 5-10 minutes, or as long as you feel comfortable.
- To get out of the posture, carefully bend your knees and roll back to a sitting position.

Tips to help you perform Chair Legs Up the Wall Pose in the right way:

- Make sure that your back is flat against the mat or blanket.
- If you have any lower back discomfort, you might tuck a rolled-up towel under your lower back for support.
- You may also lay a cushion beneath your head for comfort.
- Focus on your breath and relax your mind and body.

The Chair Legs Up the Wall Pose is a terrific method to relax and de-stress. It is also an excellent posture to take before or after a yoga session. If you are seeking a technique to increase your circulation, decrease stress, and improve your general health, I invite you to try this stance.

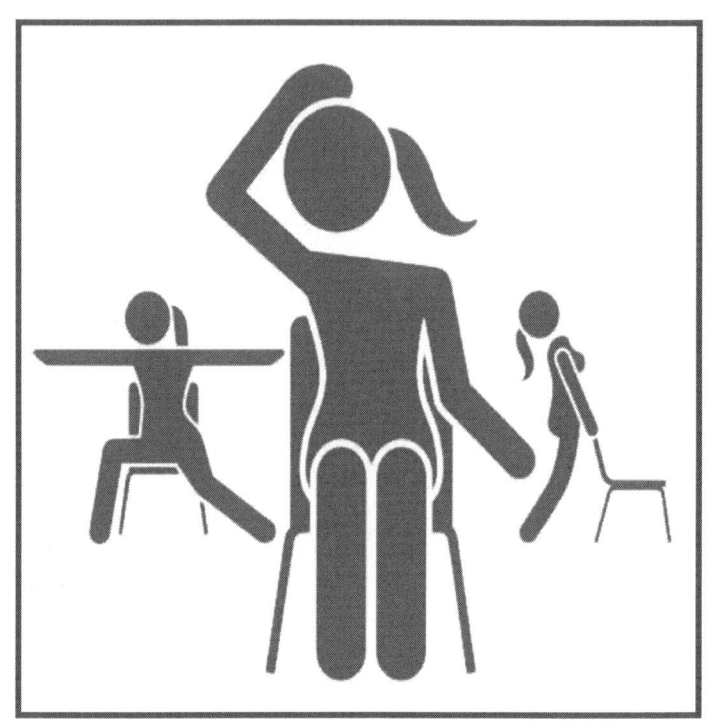

CHAPTER FOUR

The Seven (7) Best Chair Yoga Poses

1. Chair Chest Opener

Follow these Instructions to help you accomplish Chair Chest Opener exercise:

- Sit in a chair with your feet flat on the floor and your back straight.
- Place your hands behind your back, fingers interlaced.
- Inhale and gently pull your hands up, maintaining your elbows straight.
- Continue elevating your hands until you feel a slight stretch in your chest and shoulders.
- Hold the stance for 5-10 breaths, then gently drop your hands back down.

Tips to help you perform Chair Chest Opener exercise in the right way:

- If you experience any discomfort, cease the workout and contact a doctor or physical therapist.
- You may change the workout by putting your hands on the back of the chair instead of interlacing them.
- If you are unable to raise your hands up all the way, it is alright. Just go as far as you can without hurting.
- The Chair Chest Opener exercise is a terrific technique to stretch and open up the chest, shoulders, and torso. It may assist to improve posture, decrease tension, and promote flexibility.

Advantages of practicing chest opening exercises:

- They may aid in enhancing breathing.

- They may assist to reduce stress in the neck and shoulders.
- They may assist to enhance circulation.
- They may assist to alleviate tension and anxiety.
- They may assist to improve posture.

If you are seeking a strategy to enhance your general health and well-being, chest opening exercises are a terrific alternative. You may perform them at home, in the workplace, or anyplace you have a chair. So get started now and feel the advantages!

2. Forward Fold

Follow these Instructions to help you accomplish chair forward fold exercise:

- Sit on the edge of a chair with your feet flat on the floor, hip-width apart.
- Place your hands on your knees, palms down.

- Inhale and stretch your spine.
- On the exhale, fold forward from your hips, keeping your back flat and your core engaged.
- Reach your arms towards the floor, or as far as you can comfortably go.
- Keep your head down and your neck relaxed.
- Hold the stretch for 30 seconds to 1 minute, or as long as is comfortable.
- To come up, inhale and gently straighten your back.

Here are some suggestions for executing the chair forward fold safely:

- If you experience any discomfort in your back, knees, or shoulders, pause and alter the stance.
- You may also bend your knees slightly to make the stretch more accessible.

- If you are unable to reach the floor, put your hands on your shins or thighs.
- Breathe deeply and relax into the stretch.

Advantages of executing the chair forward fold:

- Improves flexibility of the hamstrings, calves, and back muscles.
- Helps to reduce stress in the back and neck.
- Promotes relaxation and stress reduction.
- Improves circulation.
- Stimulates the digestive system.
- Can help to decrease headaches.

The chair forward fold is an excellent technique to stretch your hamstrings, calves, and back muscles. It may also assist to increase your flexibility and range of motion. If you are new to yoga or stretching, start with a shorter hold and progressively increase the duration as you get more comfortable.

3. Side Bends

Follow these Instructions to help you accomplish chair side bends:

- Sit on a firm chair with your feet flat on the floor hip-width apart.
- Place your hands behind your head, fingers interlaced.
- Engage your core and maintain your back straight.
- Slowly bend to the right side, maintaining your hips and shoulders square.
- Pause for a second at the bottom of the curve, then gently return to the starting position.
- Repeat on the left side.
- Do 10-15 repetitions on each side.

Here are some guidelines for performing chair side bends safely:

- Don't bend too much to the side, since this might put tension on your back.
- Keep your core engaged throughout the workout.
- Don't arch your back.
- If you suffer any discomfort, quit the workout.

Chair side bends are a terrific exercise for targeting the oblique muscles, which are positioned on the sides of your belly. Strong oblique muscles may assist improve your posture and balance, and they can also help you burn calories and reduce weight.

However, it is vital to remember that side bends are not the perfect workout for everyone. If you have any back problems, you should avoid this activity. There are additional workouts that might help you target the oblique muscles without placing stress on your back.

Here are several alternatives to chair side bends:

- Plank with side twist
- Russian twists
- Bird dog Side plank with reach
- Hanging leg raises

If you are new to exercising, it is usually a good idea to chat to your doctor before beginning any new regimen.

4. Neck Stretches

Follow these Instructions to help you accomplish chair neck stretches:

- **Chin to chest stretch:** Sit up straight in your chair with your shoulders relaxed. Slowly drop your chin towards your chest until you feel a stretch on the back of your neck. Hold the stretch for 10 seconds, then gently return to the starting position. Repeat 3 times.

- **Ear to shoulder stretch:** Sit up straight in your chair with your shoulders relaxed. Gently tilt your head to one side, moving your ear nearer your shoulder. Hold the stretch for 10 seconds, then gently return to the starting position. Repeat on the opposite side.

- **Neck rotation stretch:** Sit up straight in your chair with your shoulders relaxed. Slowly twist your head clockwise, being careful to maintain your chin tucked in. Hold the stretch for 10 seconds, then gently twist your head counterclockwise. Repeat 3 times.

- **Neck side bend stretch:** Sit up straight in your chair with your shoulders relaxed.

Gently tilt your head to one side, keeping your chin tucked in. Hold the stretch for 10 seconds, then gently return to the starting position. Repeat on the opposite side.

- **Neck extension stretch:** Sit up straight in your chair with your shoulders relaxed. Slowly tilt your head back, staring up at the ceiling. Hold the stretch for 10 seconds, then gently return to the starting position.

You may practice these stretches once or twice a day, or anytime you feel your neck growing stiff. It is vital to listen to your body and stop if you feel any discomfort.

Here are some other recommendations for practicing chair neck stretches:

- Breathe deeply and gently during the stretch.
- Don't force the stretch.

- If you experience any discomfort, stop immediately.
- Hold each stretch for 10 seconds.
- Repeat each stretch 3 times.
- Be careful to relax your shoulders and neck muscles during the stretch.

5. Backbend

Follow these Instructions to help you accomplish Chair Backbend exercise:

- Sit on a firm chair with your feet level on the floor and your back straight.
- Place your hands on the back of the chair, shoulder-width apart.
- Inhale and arch your back, raising your chest and head up.
- Look up towards the ceiling and hold the stance for 5-10 breaths.
- Exhale and gently release back to the beginning position.

Here are some suggestions for completing the Chair Backbend exercise safely:

- Don't push the stance if you feel any discomfort.
- If you are new to backbends, start with a softer variant, such as the sitting backbend with a wrapped towel behind your lower back.
- Be cautious to warm up your body before completing any backbends.
- Come out of the stance softly and gradually.

Here are various variants of the Chair Backbend exercise:

- For a more hard variant, consider putting your hands on the floor behind you, shoulder-width apart.

- You may also try putting a wrapped towel behind your lower back for support.

The Chair Backbend exercise is an excellent technique to stretch your back, shoulders, and chest. It may also assist to enhance your posture and flexibility.

If you are new to backbends, make cautious to start softly and progressively increase the severity of the position as you grow more flexible.

6. Seated Twist

Follow these Instructions to help you accomplish chair sitting twist exercise:

- Sit on a solid chair with your feet level on the floor and your knees bent at a 90-degree angle.
- Place your hands on your hips, with your fingers pointing down.

- Slowly rotate your upper body to the right, maintaining your spine long and your shoulders relaxed.
- Look over your right shoulder as you twist.
- Hold the twist for a few seconds, then gently return to the center.
- Repeat on the opposite side.

Here are some suggestions for completing the chair sitting twist exercise safely and effectively:

- Don't push the twist if you feel any discomfort.
- Keep your core engaged throughout the workout.
- Breathe deeply and evenly as you twist.
- Do not twist your neck.
- Start with a few repetitions and progressively increase the number as you gain stronger.

Advantages of practicing the chair sitting twist exercise:

- Improves flexibility and range of motion in the spine
- Helps to ease back pain Improves digestion
- Tones the abdominal muscles
- Helps to cleanse the organs
- Reduces stress

The chair sitting twist exercise is an effective approach to enhance your flexibility and range of motion in your spine. It may also assist to reduce back pain and improve digestion. If you are new to exercising, it is usually a good idea to chat to your doctor before beginning any new regimen.

7. *Spinal Twist*

Follow these Instructions to help you accomplish chair spinal twist:

- Sit in a chair with your feet flat on the floor and your back straight.
- Place your right hand on the back of the chair behind you.
- Inhale and stretch your spine.
- Exhale and rotate your body to the right, keeping your shoulders relaxed.
- Rest your left hand on your thigh or on the outside of your right leg.
- Hold the twist for 5-10 breaths, or as long as it is comfortable.
- To emerge from the posture, inhale and stretch your spine.
- Exhale and twist back to center.
- Repeat on the opposite side.

Here are some pointers for completing a chair spinal twist safely:

- Don't push the twist. If you experience any discomfort, stop.
- Keep your shoulders relaxed and low.

- Breathe deeply during the position.
- If you have any neck or back concerns, consult your doctor before attempting this posture.

Advantages of practicing chair spinal twist exercises:

- Improves spinal mobility.
- Stretches the neck, chest, shoulders, upper and lower back.
- Opens up the hips.
- Improves posture.
- Can assist to ease neck and upper back discomfort.
- Reduces tension and anxiety.
- Improves digestion.
- Promotes relaxation.

The chair spinal twist is an effective approach to promote spinal mobility, extend the neck, chest, shoulders, and upper back, and open up the hips.

The Six (6) Breathing Yoga Exercises For Seniors

1. Deep Breathing

Follow these Instructions to help you accomplish chair deep breathing exercises:

- Find a comfy chair to sit in. Make sure your back is straight and your feet are flat on the floor.
- Place one hand on your chest and the other slightly below your rib cage. This will enable you to feel your diaphragm move as you breathe.
- Close your eyes and relax your body.
- Inhale gently through your nose, feeling your tummy rise against your palm.
- Hold your breath for a little time.
- Exhale gently through your lips, feeling your stomach collapse.
- Repeat steps 4-6 for 5-10 minutes.

Here are some recommendations for practicing chair deep breathing exercises:

- Breathe deeply and gently. Don't force your breath.
- Focus on your breath and the movement of your diaphragm.
- Relax your body and get rid of any stress.
- If you feel your thoughts drifting, gently bring it back to your breath.

Advantages of chair deep breathing exercises:

- Improves sleep quality
- Reduces anxiety and depression
- Lowers blood pressure
- Improves attention and concentration
- Boosts the immune system
- Relieves discomfort

Chair deep breathing exercises can be done anywhere, at any time. They are an effective method to reduce stress, enhance your mood, and raise your energy levels.

3. Nadi Shodhana

Chair Nadi Shodhana is a version of the conventional Nadi Shodhana pranayama, or alternating nostril breathing, that may be done while seated in a chair. It is a simple yet powerful practice that may help to relax the mind and body, increase attention, and decrease stress.

Follow these Instructions to help you accomplish Chair Nadi Shodhana:

- Sit in a comfortable chair with your back straight and your feet flat on the floor.
- Place your right index finger on your right nostril and your right ring finger on your left nostril.

- Inhale gently and deeply through your left nostril.
- Close your left nostril with your ring finger and exhale gently through your right nose.
- Inhale gently and deeply via your right nostril.
- Close your right nostril with your index finger and exhale gently through your left nose.
- Continue this pattern for 5-10 minutes, or for as long as you feel comfortable.

If you are new to Nadi Shodhana, you may wish to start with a shorter length of time, such as 3-5 minutes. You may also try shutting one nostril for a few seconds at a time, before switching to the other nose.

As you breathe, concentrate on the sensation of the air passing through your nose. You may also want to concentrate on your breath moving to other regions of your body, such as your chest, abdomen, and head.

If you feel your thoughts drifting, gently bring your focus back to your breath.

Nadi Shodhana is a safe and moderate workout that may be done by individuals of all ages and fitness levels. However, if you have any health problems, it is always wise to speak with your doctor before beginning any new fitness regimen.

Advantages of Nadi Shodhana:

- It may assist to soothe the mind and body.
- It may increase attention and concentration.
- It may alleviate tension and anxiety.
- It may increase sleep quality.
- It may enhance the immune system.
- It may assist to manage blood pressure and heart rate.

4. Meditation for Seniors

Follow these Instructions to help you accomplish chair meditation for seniors:

- Find a comfy chair to sit in. Make sure that your back is straight and your feet are flat on the floor.
- Close your eyes and take a few deep breaths. Focus on your breath as it enters and departs your body.
- As you breathe, assess your body for any places of tightness. Notice where you feel tension or pain.
- With each breath, allow those places to relax. Let go of any tension or stress that you are hanging onto.
- Continue to breathe deeply and concentrate on relaxation. You may wish to repeat a mantra or affirmation to yourself, such as "I am calm and relaxed" or "I am at peace."
- When you are ready, open your eyes and gently come back to the present time.

Here are some extra recommendations for chair meditation for seniors:

- Start with a brief meditation, such as 5 or 10 minutes. Gradually expand the time of your meditation as you feel more comfortable with it.
- If you have any health problems, speak to your doctor before beginning a new meditation practice.
- Find a peaceful area to meditate where you will not be interrupted.
- Dress comfortably and wear loose-fitting clothes.
- If you need to, use a cushion or pillow to support your back or legs.
- Be patient with yourself and don't become disappointed if your mind wanders during meditation. Just slowly return your focus back to your breath.

Here are some alternative chair meditation techniques that you might try:

- **Shoulder rolls:** Slowly move your shoulders forward and then backward. Repeat 5 times.
- **Neck stretches:** Gently tilt your head to the right, then to the left. Repeat 5 times.
- **Arm circles:** Make little circles with your arms, first clockwise and then counterclockwise. Repeat 5 repeats each way.
- **Leg stretches:** Reach down and touch your toes, keeping your back straight. Hold for a few seconds, then release.
- **Chest opener:** Bring your arms up above and clasp your hands together. Gently draw your arms apart, exposing your chest. Hold for a few seconds, then release.

Chair meditation is an effective technique for elders to relax and de-stress. It may also assist to enhance sleep, relieve discomfort, and raise mood. If you are seeking a strategy to enhance your well-being, chair meditation is a fantastic choice to investigate.

5. Mindfulness Meditation

Follow these Instructions to help you accomplish chair mindfulness meditation exercise:

- Find a comfy chair to sit in. Your back should be upright, but not rigid. Your feet should be flat on the floor.
- Close your eyes or look lightly at a point on the floor in front of you.
- Bring your focus to your breath. Notice the rise and fall of your chest and abdomen as you breathe in and out.
- If your mind wanders, gently bring it back to your breath. Don't criticize yourself for becoming sidetracked. Just keep returning your focus back to your breath.
- Continue to sit with your concentration on your breath for 5-10 minutes.

- When you're ready, open your eyes and take a few calm, deep breaths.

Here are some extra guidelines for practicing a chair mindfulness meditation exercise:

- If you feel yourself becoming fidgety, consider altering your posture or moving your weight.
- If you experience any discomfort, consider altering your position or taking a break.
- If you start to feel tired, open your eyes or gently shake your head.
- Be patient with yourself. It takes time and effort to master the skill of mindfulness meditation.

Advantages of chair mindfulness meditation:

- Reduces stress and anxiety
- Improves attention and concentration
- Helps to manage pain

- Improves sleep quality
- Boosts mood
- Increases self-awareness
- Promotes relaxation

If you are new to mindfulness meditation, I suggest beginning with a brief practice of 5-10 minutes. You may progressively extend the time of your practice as you feel more comfortable with it.

6. Guided Meditation

Follow these Instructions to help you accomplish chair guided meditation:

- Find a comfy chair to sit in. Make sure that your back is straight and your feet are flat on the floor.
- Close your eyes and take a few deep breaths. Notice the sensation of the air as it enters and exits your lungs.

- Bring your focus to your body. Notice any regions of tension or tightness. Gently relax these regions.
- Focus on your breath. Notice the rise and fall of your chest as you breathe in and out.
- If your mind wanders, gently bring it back to your breath. Don't condemn yourself for having thoughts, simply let them go and return back to your breath.
- Continue to meditate for 5-10 minutes. When you're through, take a few deep breaths and open your eyes.

Here are some extra suggestions for chair guided meditation:

- Find a peaceful area where you won't be bothered.
- Wear comfy clothes.
- If you experience any discomfort, modify your position until you're comfortable.

- If you fall asleep, that's acceptable. Just slowly wake yourself up and start over.
- With frequent practice, you'll discover that chair guided meditation may assist you to relax, decrease tension, and enhance your general well-being.

Here is a guided meditation script that you may follow:

- Find a comfy chair to sit in. Close your eyes and take a few deep breaths.
- As you breathe in, repeat to yourself, "I am breathing in peace." As you breathe out, repeat to yourself, "I am breathing out stress."
- Continue to breathe in serenity and breathe out worry for a few minutes.
- Now, direct your attention to your body. Notice any regions of tension or tightness. Gently relax these regions.

- Focus on your breath again. Notice the rise and fall of your chest as you breathe in and out.
- If your mind wanders, gently bring it back to your breath. Don't condemn yourself for having thoughts, simply let them go and return back to your breath.
- Continue to meditate for 5-10 minutes. When you're through, take a few deep breaths and open your eyes.

You may discover many additional guided meditation scripts online or in books. Choose one that you find peaceful and that connects with you.

With frequent practice, you'll discover that chair guided meditation may be a beneficial approach to decrease stress, enhance your mood, and raise your general well-being.

Sixteen (16) Chair Yoga Cardio Exercise For Weight Loss

1. Chair Yoga Nidra

Chair Yoga Nidra is a sort of yoga nidra that may be done while sitting in a chair. It is a strong technique for relaxation and stress alleviation, and it may also be used to promote sleep, decrease anxiety, and increase creativity.

Follow these Instructions to help you accomplish Chair Yoga Nidra:

- Find a peaceful area where you will not be bothered. Sit in a comfortable chair with your back straight and your feet flat on the floor.
- Close your eyes and take a few deep breaths. As you breathe in, repeat to yourself, "I am breathing in relaxation." As you breathe out, repeat to yourself, "I am breathing out tension."

- Bring your consciousness to your body. Notice any regions of tension or tightness. With each breath, allow those places to relax.
- Scan your body from head to toe, paying attention to each area. Notice the weight of your body on the chair, the feelings in your skin, and the movement of your breath.
- Now, pretend that you are sinking into the chair. Let go of any attempt to keep oneself upright. Allow your body to feel heavy and relaxed.
- Continue to breathe deeply and relax your body. As you do, listen to the sound of your breath. Notice the rise and fall of your chest and tummy.
- Now, bring your awareness to your thoughts. Notice any ideas that enter into your head. With each inhalation, let those ideas go.
- Continue to concentrate on your breath and the current moment. Allow yourself to be entirely relaxed.

- When you are ready, gently open your eyes. Take a few seconds to acclimatize to the light.
- You may practice Chair Yoga Nidra for as long as you desire. 20 minutes is a decent beginning point, but you may progressively extend the duration as you feel more familiar with the exercise.

Here are some ideas for doing Chair Yoga Nidra:

- Find a peaceful area where you will not be bothered.
- Wear comfy clothes.
- If you have any injuries, adapt the position to be comfortable for you.
- If you fall asleep, that's acceptable. Just slowly wake yourself up and continue with the exercise.
- Be patient with yourself and don't become disappointed if you don't understand it right

away. With consistent practice, you will become more comfortable and focused.

2. Chair arm circles

Follow these Instructions to help you accomplish chair arm circles exercise:

- Sit on a firm chair with your back straight and your feet flat on the floor.
- Hold your arms out at your sides, parallel to the floor, with your palms facing down.
- Make little circles with your arms, keeping your shoulders relaxed and your elbows slightly bent.
- Inhale as you create circles ahead and exhale as you make circles backward.
- Continue for 30 seconds to 1 minute, or as long as you comfortably can.

Here are some pointers for performing chair arm circles:

- Keep your core engaged throughout the workout.
- Don't let your shoulders slump up.
- If your arms start to feel fatigued, lower the size of the circles.
- If you experience any discomfort, cease the activity and contact with your doctor or physical therapist.

Advantages of chair arm circles exercise include:

- Warming up the shoulders, arms, chest, and back.
- Improving range of motion in the shoulders.
- Toning the muscles in the shoulders and arms.
- Reducing stress and tension.

If you are new to exercising, start with a few repetitions and progressively increase the number as you gain stronger. You may also practice chair arm circles as part of a warm-up or cool-down regimen.

3. Chair shoulder shrugs

Follow these Instructions to help you accomplish chair shoulder shrugs:

- Sit on a firm chair with your feet level on the floor and your back straight.
- Place your hands on the edge of the chair behind you, shoulder-width apart.
- Keep your elbows straight and your core engaged.
- Shrug your shoulders up towards your ears, as high as you can without moving your upper body off the chair.
- Hold for a second, then gently drop your shoulders back down.
- Repeat for 10-15 repetitions.

Here are some suggestions for executing chair shoulder shrugs securely and effectively:

- Keep your core engaged throughout the workout to avoid your back from rounding.
- Don't elevate your upper body off the chair when you shrug your shoulders.
- Don't utilize too much weight, since this might create stress on your shoulders.
- If you suffer any discomfort, quit the workout immediately.

Chair shoulder shrugs are an excellent approach to target the trapezius muscles, which are responsible for lifting and lowering the shoulders. They may also assist to improve posture and alleviate shoulder strain.

Here are various variants of the chair shoulder shrug exercise:

- You may use dumbbells or a barbell instead of your hands on the chair.
- You may complete the exercise standing up, with your feet shoulder-width apart and your core engaged.
- You may add a twist to the workout by shrugging your shoulders up and to the sides.

No matter the variant you select, be careful to execute the exercise with perfect form to prevent injury.

4. Chair chest openers

Follow these Instructions to help you accomplish chair chest openers exercise:

- Sit in a chair with your feet flat on the floor and your back straight.
- Place your hands on the back of the chair, shoulder-width apart.
- Inhale and gently lean back, keeping your shoulders down and your chest open.
- Hold the posture for a few breaths, then exhale and return to the beginning position.

Here are some pointers for practicing the chair chest openers exercise:

- If you feel any discomfort in your back, pause and alter the position by leaning back less.
- You may also drape a wrapped towel or blanket behind your lower back for support.

- Breathe deeply and evenly throughout the position.

Here are various variants of the chair chest openers exercise:

- You may stretch your arms upwards instead of laying them on the back of the chair.
- You may also interlace your fingers behind your back and bring your arms back.
- If you are more flexible, you might try reclining back with your arms outstretched in front of you.

The chair chest openers exercise is an excellent technique to expand your chest, shoulders, and back. It may help to improve your posture, decrease stress, and stimulate your circulation. If you are new to yoga, it is a good idea to start with this posture and progressively work your way up to more strenuous versions.

5. Chair twists

Chair twists are a terrific workout for developing your core muscles, particularly your obliques. Here are the instructions on how to accomplish it:

- Sit on a firm chair with your feet level on the floor and your back straight.
- Place your hands behind your head, with your elbows bent and your fingers interlaced.
- Slowly rotate your body to the right, bringing your right elbow towards your left knee.
- Hold for a second, then return to the starting position.
- Repeat on the opposite side.
- You may complete 10-15 repetitions on each side, or as many as you can comfortably accomplish.

Here are some pointers for executing chair twists safely and effectively:

- Keep your back straight throughout the workout.
- Don't twist too much, since this might put tension on your back.
- Breathe naturally while you complete the workout.
- If you experience any discomfort, discontinue the workout and contact your doctor.

Advantages of performing chair twists:

- Strengthens your core muscles
- Improves your balance
- Helps to decrease back pain
- Improves your posture
- Burns calories
- Tones your waistline

Chair twists are an effective workout that you can perform anywhere, even if you have restricted mobility. They are a low-impact workout, so they are also easy on your joints.

6. Chair arm rises

Follow these Instructions to help you accomplish chair arm raises:

- Sit on a firm chair with your feet level on the floor and your back straight.
- Hold a dumbbell in each hand, with your palms facing up and your arms resting at your sides.
- Slowly lift your arms out to the sides, keeping your elbows slightly bent.
- Raise your arms till they are parallel to the floor, or as high as you can comfortably go.
- Pause for a minute, then gently drop your arms back to the starting position.
- Repeat 10-12 times, or as many times as you can comfortably accomplish.

Here are some guidelines for performing chair arm lifts safely:

- Use a weight that is demanding but not overly heavy. You should be able to execute 10-12 repetitions with proper technique.
- Keep your back straight and your core engaged throughout the workout.
- Don't swing your arms. The movement should be regulated and fluid.
- If you suffer any discomfort, quit the workout immediately.

Here are several variants of chair arm lifts that you might try:

- Front raises: Instead of extending your arms out to the sides, raise them in front of you.
- Bent-over raises: Bend forward at the waist, keeping your back straight, and lift your arms out to the sides.

- Lateral raises with resistance band: Attach a resistance band to a strong item over your head. Hold the ends of the band in each hand, with your palms facing down. Raise your arms out to the sides, keeping the band tight.

Chair arm rises are an excellent approach to strengthen your shoulders and upper arms. They may be done at home with minimal equipment, making them a practical and accessible workout for everyone.

7. Chair leg raises

Follow these Instructions to help you accomplish chair leg lifts:

- Sit at the edge of a solid chair with your feet flat on the floor.
- Lean back slightly so that your back is not contacting the chair backrest.

- Keep your core engaged and your back straight.
- Slowly pull one leg up, keeping your knee straight.
- Lift your leg as high as you can without straining your back.
- Hold the posture for a few seconds, then gently drop your leg back down.
- Repeat steps 4-6 with the opposite leg.
- You may complete 10-15 repetitions of each leg. If you are a novice, you may start with less repetitions and progressively increase the number as you gain stronger.

Here are some pointers for performing chair leg lifts:

- Keep your core engaged throughout the workout. This will assist to avoid back discomfort.
- Don't elevate your leg too high. If you feel any discomfort in your back, drop your leg.

- Breathe regularly during the activity.

Advantages of performing chair leg lifts:

- Strengthens the core and lower abs.
- Improves balance and coordination.
- Helps to avoid back discomfort.
- Improves circulation.
- Burns calories.

If you are searching for a method to get a nice exercise without having to leave your chair, chair leg lifts are a terrific alternative. Just be careful to perform them properly to prevent harm.

8. Chair knee tucks

Follow these Instructions to help you accomplish chair knee tucks:

- Sit in a firm chair with your hands on the edge of the seat for support.

- Lean back slightly so that your back is not contacting the back of the chair.
- Extend your legs out in front of you, keeping your knees straight.
- As you exhale, bend your knees and pull your feet closer to your chest.
- Keep your back straight and your core engaged throughout the action.
- Hold for a second at the peak of the contraction, then gently drop your legs back to the starting position.
- Repeat for the appropriate amount of repetitions.

Here are some pointers for performing chair knee tucks:

- Keep your core engaged throughout the action. This will assist to protect your back and avoid injuries.
- Don't round your back. Keep your back straight and your shoulders relaxed.

- If you are unable to maintain your legs straight, bend them slightly.
- Start with a few repetitions and progressively increase the number as you gain stronger.

Here are several variants of chair knee tucks that you might try:

- To make the exercise more demanding, consider completing it without using your hands for support.
- You may also try completing the exercise with your feet raised on a bench or step.
- If you are unable to accomplish the entire range of motion, you may execute the exercise with your knees bent.

Chair knee tucks are a wonderful workout for training your core muscles, including your abs, hip flexors, and quadriceps. They can also assist to enhance your balance and coordination.

9. Chair hip circles

Follow these Instructions to help you accomplish chair hip circles:

- Sit on a chair with your feet level on the floor and your knees bent at a 90-degree angle.
- Place your hands on your thighs for support.
- Slowly rotate your hips in a circular circle, being careful to maintain your back straight.
- Continue twisting your hips for 10-15 repetitions.
- Reverse the direction and spin your hips in a counterclockwise circle for 10-15 repetitions.
- Repeat steps 3-5 2-3 times.

Here are some pointers for performing chair hip circles:

- Keep your core engaged throughout the workout.

- Don't let your shoulders slump forward.
- If you experience any discomfort, quit the workout.

Advantages of chair hip circles include:

- Increased range of motion in the hips
- Reduced hip pain
- Improved flexibility
- Strengthened core muscles
- Improved balance

If you are new to exercising, start with a few repetitions and gradually increase the amount of repetitions as you gain stronger. You may also practice chair hip circles as part of a warm-up or cool-down exercise.

10. Chair hamstring stretch

Follow these Instructions to help you accomplish sitting hamstring stretch:

- Sit on the edge of a chair with your feet flat on the floor.
- Straighten one leg out in front of you, keeping your heel on the floor and your toes pointing up.
- Bend the second leg at the knee and lay the foot of that leg flat on the floor next to your first leg.
- Reach forward and hold the foot of your outstretched leg with your hand.
- Gently move your heel towards your buttock until you feel a stretch at the back of your leg.
- Keep your back straight and your core engaged.
- Hold the stretch for 30 seconds.
- Repeat on the opposite side.

Here are some suggestions for practicing a sitting hamstring stretch:

- Don't force the stretch. If you experience any discomfort, stop immediately.
- Keep your back straight during the stretch.
- If you have tight hamstrings, you may not be able to straighten your leg fully at the beginning. That's alright. Just bend your leg as much as you can and progressively expand the range of motion over time.
- You may also execute this stretch using a resistance band. Wrap the band around the ball of your foot and grasp the ends of the band in your palms. Gently pull the band towards you to increase the stretch.

The sitting hamstring stretch is an excellent approach to develop flexibility in your hamstrings. Hamstrings are the muscles at the back of your thigh that help you bend your knees and straighten your hips. Tight hamstrings may make it difficult to accomplish regular tasks, such as walking, jogging, and getting up from a chair. Stretching your hamstrings frequently may assist to increase your flexibility and range of motion, and minimize discomfort and stiffness.

11. Chair calf stretch

Follow these Instructions to help you accomplish chair calf stretch:

- Sit on the edge of a chair with your feet flat on the floor and your knees bent at a 90-degree angle.
- Place one hand on the chair for balance.
- Reach forward with the other hand and hold the toes of your extended leg.
- Gently draw your toes towards your shinbone until you feel a stretch at the back of your calf.
- Hold the stretch for 30-60 seconds.
- Repeat on the opposite leg.

Here are some pointers for performing a chair calf stretch:

- Make sure your back is straight and your core is engaged during the stretch.
- Don't bounce or push the stretch.
- If you experience any discomfort, discontinue the stretch immediately.

You can also perform a chair calf stretch with a towel or resistance band. To accomplish this, repeat the identical steps above, but instead of grabbing your toes, loop the towel or band around your foot and hold the ends of the towel or band in your hands.

Calf stretches are an effective method to enhance your flexibility and range of motion. They may also assist to avoid calf injuries. If you experience any pain or discomfort, discontinue the stretch immediately and contact a doctor or physical therapist.

12. Chair squat

Follow these Instructions to help you accomplish chair squats:

- Stand in front of a solid chair with your feet hip-width apart and your toes pointed forward.
- Place your hands on your hips or in front of you for balance.
- Slowly bend your knees and drop your body down toward the chair, maintaining your back straight and your core engaged.
- Stop when your thighs are parallel to the floor or slightly lower.
- Push through your heels to stand back up to the starting position.

Here are some pointers for performing chair squats correctly:

- Keep your back straight and your core engaged throughout the action.

- Don't allow your knees to go beyond your toes.
- Don't lean forward or backward.
- If you're suffering discomfort, stop and alter the activity.

You may start with 10-15 reps and progressively increase the amount of repetitions as you grow stronger. You may also add weight to the workout by holding dumbbells or a weight plate in front of you.

Here are various versions of chair squats that you might try:

- **Standing chair squats:** This is the simplest variant of the chair squat.
- **Wall chair squats:** Stand facing a wall with your feet hip-width apart and your toes touching the wall. Slowly bend your knees and drop your body down toward the wall,

maintaining your back straight and your core engaged.

- **Single-leg chair squats:** Stand in front of a chair with your feet shoulder-width apart. Lift one leg off the ground and bend your other leg to drop your body down toward the chair. Keep your back straight and your core engaged.
- **Chair step-ups:** Stand in front of a chair with your feet hip-width apart. Step up onto the chair with one leg and then step back down with the same leg. Repeat with the opposite leg.

Chair squats are a fantastic workout for beginners and persons with restricted mobility. They may assist to strengthen your legs, glutes, and core.

13. Chair lunge

Follow these Instructions to help you accomplish chair lunge exercise:

- Stand facing a solid chair with your feet hip-width apart. Place your hands on the back of the chair for support.
- Step forward with your right leg, keeping your left leg behind you.
- Bend both knees, lowering your body until your right thigh is parallel to the floor. Your back knee should be close to the floor, but not touching.
- Push off with your right foot to return to the starting position.
- Repeat on the opposite side.

Here are some pointers for executing chair lunges safely and effectively:

- Keep your back straight and your core engaged throughout the workout.

- Don't allow your front knee to go beyond your toes.
- If you experience any discomfort, stop and adapt the workout.
- You may start with 10-12 reps on each side and progressively increase the amount of repetitions as you grow stronger. You may also add weight to the workout by carrying dumbbells in your hands.

Advantages of practicing chair lunges:

- They work the muscles in your legs, including your quadriceps, hamstrings, and glutes.
- They may assist to enhance your balance and coordination.
- They may assist to improve your core muscles.
- They may assist to alleviate lower back discomfort.

- If you are new to exercising, it is usually a good idea to chat to your doctor before beginning any new regimen.

14. Chair push-ups

Follow these Instructions to help you accomplish chair push-ups:

- Stand in front of a strong chair with armrests.
- Place your hands on the armrests, shoulder-width apart.
- Bend your knees slightly and step back until your body is in a plank posture with your arms outstretched.
- Make sure your back is straight and your core is engaged.
- Slowly lower your body until your chest hits the chair.
- Push yourself back up to the starting position.

Here are some suggestions for performing chair push-ups:

- Keep your core engaged throughout the workout.
- Don't let your back slump.
- Don't lock your elbows at the apex of the action.
- If you're struggling, you may position your feet closer to the chair.
- As you gain strength, you can move your feet farther away from the chair.

Here are various versions of chair push-ups that you may try:

- **Incline chair push-ups:** Place your feet on a higher surface, such as a table or a bench. This will make the activity easier.
- **Decline chair push-ups:** Place your feet on the floor and your hands on a lower surface,

such as a step or a stool. This will make the activity more tough.

- **One-arm chair push-ups:** Place one hand on the chair and the other hand on the floor. This will work your core even more.

Chair push-ups are an excellent workout for individuals of all fitness levels. They are a low-impact approach to train your chest, triceps, and core.

15. Chair planks

A chair plank is a modified form of the regular plank that is gentler on the wrists and shoulders. It is a fantastic workout for beginners or persons with injuries.

Follow these Instructions to help you accomplish chair plank:

- Stand in front of a strong chair and lay your forearms on the seat, shoulder-width apart.

- Step your feet back so that your body forms a straight line from your head to your heels.
- Engage your core muscles and clench your glutes.
- Hold this posture for as long as you can, breathing normally.
- To get out of the posture, carefully move your feet forward and drop your forearms to the floor.

Here are some suggestions for performing a chair plank:

- Keep your body in a straight line from your head to your heels.
- Don't allow your hips to sink or your back arch.
- Engage your core muscles and clench your glutes.
- If you find it too difficult to maintain the posture for a long period, start with a shorter duration and gradually increase it.

Here are various versions of the chair plank:

- To make it more tough, elevate one leg off the floor at a time.
- To make it simpler, put your hands on the side of the chair instead of the seat.
- You may also try performing a chair plank with your knees bent.

The chair plank is an excellent technique to improve your core muscles. It might also assist to enhance your posture and balance.

16. Chair mountain climbers

Chair mountain climbers are a modified form of the classic mountain climbers workout that makes it simpler for novices or persons with restricted mobility. To do chair mountain climbers, you will need a strong chair.

Here are the steps:

- Stand facing the chair with your feet shoulder-width apart.
- Place your hands on the edge of the chair, a little wider than shoulder-width apart.
- Lower your body down into a plank posture, maintaining your back straight and your core engaged.
- Bring your right knee up towards your chest, keeping your left leg stretched behind you.
- Return your right leg to the beginning position and repeat with your left knee.
- Continue alternating between sides, pushing each knee up towards your chest as rapidly as you can.

Here are some pointers for doing chair mountain climbers:

- Keep your core engaged throughout the workout.

- Don't let your back slump.
- If you're suffering discomfort in your wrists, you may put your hands on the floor instead of the chair.
- Start with a few sets of 10-15 repetitions and progressively increase the amount of sets and reps as you gain stronger.

Advantages of doing chair mountain climbers:

- They assist to develop your core muscles, which are vital for maintaining excellent posture and reducing back problems.
- They work your leg muscles, particularly your quadriceps, hamstrings, and calves.
- They may assist to enhance your cardiovascular health.
- They are a low-impact workout, making them an excellent alternative for persons with joint problems.

CHAPTER FIVE

How To Avoid Injury And Optimize The Benefits Of A Chair Yoga Practice

If you want to avoid injuries and optimize the benefits of chair yoga, you need to follow these tips accordingly:

1. Start softly and progressively raise the intensity of your practice over time. Don't attempt to do too much too quickly, or you're more likely to be harmed.

2. Listen to your body and adapt positions as required. If a position is causing discomfort, pause and attempt a new one.

3. Use props to support your body. A block or rolled-up towel may be useful for getting into and out of postures, and for giving support for your back, neck, or shoulders.

4. Breathe deeply and deliberately throughout your practice. This will help you relax and concentrate on your body, and it will also assist to avoid injury.

5. Warm up before you start your practice and cool down afterwards. This will assist to prepare your body for activities and avoid discomfort.

6. Stay hydrated. Drink lots of water before, during, and after your practice.

7. Find a competent teacher. If you're new to chair yoga, it's a good idea to locate a certified teacher who can help you learn the postures and adjustments safely.

Optimizing the advantages of practicing your chair yoga:

1. Practice frequently. The more you practice, the more advantages you'll enjoy. Aim for at least 30 minutes of chair yoga 2-3 times per week.

2. Find a peaceful spot to practice where you won't be disturbed. This will enable you to concentrate on your practice and calm your thoughts.

3. Wear comfortable attire that enables you to move freely. You may also wish to wear socks to protect your feet from sliding.

4. Set aside some time for yourself to relax and enjoy your practice. Chair yoga is a terrific method to de-stress and enhance your general well-being.

How To Make Easy Food Choices That Will Increase Your Flexibility, Lower Your Inflammation And Live A Healthier Lifestyle

The basic dietary choices that can increase flexibility and minimize inflammation are as follows:

- **Eat lots of fruits and veggies.** Fruits and vegetables are rich with vitamins, minerals, and antioxidants that are vital for joint health. They are also low in calories and fat, which might help you maintain a healthy weight. Some ideal options for joint health are berries, leafy greens, citrus fruits, and cruciferous vegetables (like broccoli and Brussels sprouts).

- **Consume fatty fish.** Fatty fish, such as salmon, tuna, and mackerel, are a strong source of omega-3 fatty acids, which have been demonstrated to lower inflammation and alleviate joint discomfort.

- **Nuts and seeds.** Nuts and seeds are a wonderful source of protein, fiber, and healthy fats. They are also an excellent source of magnesium, which is a vital element for joint health. Some healthy alternatives are almonds, walnuts, and chia seeds.

- **Whole grains.** Whole grains are a rich source of fiber, which may help to decrease inflammation. They are also an excellent source of complex carbs, which may give continuous energy throughout the day. Some healthful alternatives are brown rice, quinoa, and oats.

- **Limit processed foods.** Processed meals are generally heavy in harmful fats, sugar, and salt. These compounds may lead to inflammation and joint discomfort.

- **Drink lots of water.** Staying hydrated is vital for general health, including joint health. Water helps to lubricate the joints and clean away impurities. Aim to consume eight glasses of water every day.

- **Include spices in your diet.** Some spices, such as turmeric and ginger, have anti-inflammatory qualities. Adding these spices to your diet may help to minimize joint pain and inflammation.

It is also crucial to undertake regular exercise and maintain a healthy weight. Exercise helps to keep your joints healthy and flexible, and it may also assist to minimize inflammation. Maintaining a healthy weight might also assist to alleviate stress on your joints.

By adopting the modest dietary modifications, you can assist to enhance your flexibility and decrease inflammation in your joints. This may lead to increased joint health and pain reduction.

CONCLUSION

Chair yoga is a safe and effective technique for seniors to enhance their physical and mental health. It is a low-impact kind of exercise that may be customized to match the requirements of people.

Chair yoga may enable seniors to enhance their flexibility, strength, balance, and range of motion. It may also assist to decrease stress, anxiety, and sadness.

If you are a senior, or know a senior who is searching for a means to enhance their health, chair yoga is a terrific alternative. It is a safe and effective approach to acquire exercise and enhance your general well-being.

There Is No More Information!

Thank you for ordering this book **"Chair Yoga For Seniors Over 70"** and I hope that you like it.

If you have an experience with the book that you would want to share with me, I would highly appreciate it!

Please take a minute to write me a **"FAVORABLE REVIEW"** on the site on which you bought the book or any other online review community. By providing me the chance to gather feedback from you, you will assist to make this book better for future readers and help to broaden its reach.

To show my appreciation, I am offering a complimentary email consultation to answer

any questions you may have about this book. Maybe you're confused on a certain concept or require help understanding it better - I'm Here To Help.

To take advantage of this offer, just drop me an email at jhendersonanne@gmail.com with the title "Book Consultation" and a brief description of whatever issue you need help with. I will do my best to get back to you within 24 hours with a useful response.

Don't forget to post a review on this book.

Thank You For Making This Purchase And I Look Forward To Your Email.

BONUS SECTION

The Step By Step Guide On How To Claim The Complementary Ebooks.

1. To Claim This Book "10 WEIGHT LOSS REFRESHING SMOOTHIES"

For Kindle:

- Click Here **to get access**

For Paperback:

- Write this UrL link manually On Your Browser to get access.

https://docs.google.com/document/d/1wYuoAoAXKhi8XhQMud9987gShJEVMF6IemM-G0iVuPw/edit?usp=drivesdk

DAILY YOGA TRACKER JOURNAL

Daily Yoga

Date _____ Time Of Day _____

Intentions

Practice Notes

Before Practice

After Practice

Did I?
- ○ Meditate
- ○ Pranayama
- ○ Sun Salutation
- ○ Moon Salutation
- ○ Let Go

Daily Yoga

Date _____ Time Of Day _____

Intentions

Practice Notes

Before Practice

After Practice

Did I?

- ○ Meditate
- ○ Pranayama
- ○ Sun Salutation
- ○ Moon Salutation
- ○ Let Go

Daily Yoga

Date _____ *Time Of Day* _____

Intentions

Practice Notes

Before Practice

After Practice

Did I?

- ○ Meditate
- ○ Pranayama
- ○ Sun Salutation
- ○ Moon Salutation
- ○ Let Go

Daily Yoga

Date _____ Time Of Day _____

Intentions

Practice Notes

Before Practice

After Practice

Did I?

- ○ Meditate
- ○ Pranayama
- ○ Sun Salutation
- ○ Moon Salutation
- ○ Let Go

Daily Yoga

Date _____ Time Of Day _____

Intentions

Practice Notes

Before Practice

After Practice

Did I?
- ○ Meditate
- ○ Pranayama
- ○ Sun Salutation
- ○ Moon Salutation
- ○ Let Go

Daily Yoga

Date _____ Time Of Day _____

Intentions

Practice Notes

Before Practice

After Practice

Did I?
- ○ Meditate
- ○ Pranayama
- ○ Sun Salutation
- ○ Moon Salutation
- ○ Let Go

Daily Yoga

Date _____ Time Of Day _____

Intentions

Practice Notes

Before Practice

After Practice

Did I?

- ○ Meditate
- ○ Pranayama
- ○ Sun Salutation
- ○ Moon Salutation
- ○ Let Go

Daily Yoga

Date _____ Time Of Day _____

Intentions

Practice Notes

Before Practice

After Practice

Did I?

- ○ Meditate
- ○ Pranayama
- ○ Sun Salutation
- ○ Moon Salutation
- ○ Let Go

Daily Yoga

Date _____ Time Of Day _____

Intentions

Practice Notes

Before Practice

After Practice

Did I?

- ○ Meditate
- ○ Pranayama
- ○ Sun Salutation
- ○ Moon Salutation
- ○ Let Go

Daily Yoga

Date _____ Time Of Day _____

Intentions

Practice Notes

Before Practice

After Practice

Did I?
- ◯ Meditate
- ◯ Pranayama
- ◯ Sun Salutation
- ◯ Moon Salutation
- ◯ Let Go

Daily Yoga

Date _____ Time Of Day _____

Intentions

Practice Notes

Before Practice

After Practice

Did I?

- ○ Meditate
- ○ Pranayama
- ○ Sun Salutation
- ○ Moon Salutation
- ○ Let Go

Daily Yoga

Date _____ Time Of Day _____

Intentions

Practice Notes

Before Practice

After Practice

Did I?

- ○ Meditate
- ○ Pranayama
- ○ Sun Salutation
- ○ Moon Salutation
- ○ Let Go

Daily Yoga

Date _____ Time Of Day _____

Intentions

Practice Notes

Before Practice

After Practice

Did I?

- ○ Meditate
- ○ Pranayama
- ○ Sun Salutation
- ○ Moon Salutation
- ○ Let Go

Daily Yoga

Date _____ Time Of Day _____

Intentions

Practice Notes

Before Practice

After Practice

Did I?

- ○ Meditate
- ○ Pranayama
- ○ Sun Salutation
- ○ Moon Salutation
- ○ Let Go

Daily Yoga

Date _____ Time Of Day _____

Intentions

Practice Notes

Before Practice

After Practice

Did I?
- ○ Meditate
- ○ Pranayama
- ○ Sun Salutation
- ○ Moon Salutation
- ○ Let Go

Daily Yoga

Date _____ Time Of Day _____

Intentions

Practice Notes

Before Practice

After Practice

Did I?

- ○ Meditate
- ○ Pranayama
- ○ Sun Salutation
- ○ Moon Salutation
- ○ Let Go

Daily Yoga

Date _____ Time Of Day _____

Intentions

Practice Notes

Before Practice

After Practice

Did I?

○ Meditate
○ Pranayama
○ Sun Salutation
○ Moon Salutation
○ Let Go

Daily Yoga

Date _____ Time Of Day _____

Intentions

Practice Notes

Before Practice

After Practice

Did I?

- ○ Meditate
- ○ Pranayama
- ○ Sun Salutation
- ○ Moon Salutation
- ○ Let Go

Daily Yoga

Date _____ Time Of Day _____

Intentions

Practice Notes

Before Practice

After Practice

Did I?

- ○ Meditate
- ○ Pranayama
- ○ Sun Salutation
- ○ Moon Salutation
- ○ Let Go

Daily Yoga

Date _____ *Time Of Day* _____

Intentions

Practice Notes

Before Practice

After Practice

Did I?

- ○ Meditate
- ○ Pranayama
- ○ Sun Salutation
- ○ Moon Salutation
- ○ Let Go

Printed in Great Britain
by Amazon